# ESSENTIAL GUIDE TO BULLOUS PEMPHIGOID

## Comprehensive Insights for Diagnosis, Treatment, and Patient Care

DR. CASEY LOREN

# DISCLAIMER

This book's content is only meant to be used for general informative purposes. Although the author has taken great care to ensure the content is accurate and thorough, no warranties or assurances on the information's accuracy, correctness, or reliability are provided. It is recommended that readers employ their own judgment and discretion when applying any material found in this book to their particular situation.

The information in this book is not intended to replace professional advice, nor is the author an expert in any of the subjects covered. It is recommended that readers consult with experienced professionals regarding any particular issues or concerns.

Any name that may be mentioned or referred in this book does not imply endorsement, recommendation, or relationship on the part of the author with any person, entity, good, website, or association. These references are made only for informational purposes and are not meant to be taken as recommendations or endorsements.

The information contained in this book may cause readers to suffer loss or damage, for which the author disclaims all obligation and accountability. The only people accountable for the decisions and actions taken by readers using the information presented are themselves.

Any names, characters, companies, locations, activities, occasions, and incidents referenced in this book are either made up or the result of the author's imagination. Any likeness to real people, living or dead, or to real things is entirely coincidental.

This book's content may change at any time, without prior notice, according to the author.

The onus is on the reader to verify whether there have been any updates or revisions.

The reader accepts the conditions of this disclaimer by reading this book. Please do not read this book or use its contents if you do not agree to these terms.

**Table of Contents**

# CHAPTER 1

## OVERVIEW OF BULLOUS PEMPHIGOID

### Synopsis and Definition

Bullous pemphigoid disease (BP) is an uncommon, long-lasting autoimmune skin condition marked by huge blisters (bullae) filled with fluid that mostly occur on the skin's outer layers. The immune system accidentally targets the basement membrane, which divides the epidermis from the dermis, causing blisters. If left untreated, this illness can cause severe pain, discomfort, and even consequences. Although it can happen at any age, blood pressure usually affects older persons, particularly those over 60. Its symptoms, which include itching and urticaria (hives), can manifest in a variety of ways, from localized blistering to widespread blistering.

# Epidemiology and History

While similar blistering disorders were mentioned in medical literature as early as the 19th century, bullous pemphigoid was first documented in the 1950s. Since then, developments in immunology and dermatology have enhanced our comprehension of the pathophysiology of BP, resulting in improved diagnostic and therapeutic approaches. According to epidemiological data, blood pressure is more prevalent in the elderly; in Western nations, the prevalence is estimated to be 6-7 cases per million years. The development of BP may be influenced by variables like aging, genetic predisposition, and environmental triggers such as specific drugs or illnesses.

# Awareness Is Vital

It is important to be aware of BP for several reasons:

**Early Diagnosis**: Treatment results can be enhanced and serious consequences can be avoided with early detection and diagnosis.

- **Patient Education**: Knowledgeable people are better able to control their illness, follow their treatment regimens, and spot flare-ups early on.

- **Healthcare Provider Training**: Increased knowledge among medical professionals guarantees that they can quickly recognize symptoms, distinguish blood pressure from related disorders, and administer the right treatment.

- **Research and Advocacy**: Raising awareness encourages financing for research as well as advocacy initiatives that could result in improved medications and even cures.

# Typical Illusions

There are several false beliefs about BP, such as:

**Age Exclusivity**: Blood pressure can strike anyone at any age, although it primarily affects older persons.

**Contagiousness**: Because BP is the outcome of an autoimmune reaction, it is not communicable.

- **Simple Dermatitis**: BP needs specific care because it is more severe than eczema or typical dermatitis.

- **Uniform Presentation**: Not all patients will experience classic blistering; blood pressure can manifest in a variety of ways and to varying degrees.

# Bullous Pemphigoid Types

Based on clinical and histological characteristics, BP can be divided into several types:

The most prevalent type, **Generalised Bullous Pemphigoid**, is typified by extensive blisters.

**Localised Bullous Pemphigoid**: Usually confined to the lower legs, this condition affects just a small area.

- **Mucous Membrane Pemphigoid**: Less common, affects mucous membranes as those in the mouth and eyes.

- **Erythematous Bullous Pemphigoid**: characterized by significant inflammation and redness, but fewer blisters.

- **Nodular Pemphigoid**: Firm, itchy nodules that resemble nodular prurigo.

## Effect on Life Quality

Blood pressure has a major effect on patients' quality of life:

- **Physical Discomfort**: Pain, itching, and subsequent infections are all possible effects of blisters.

- **Emotional Distress**: Social isolation, anxiety, and despair can result from long-term medical conditions and noticeable skin lesions.

**Daily Activities**: Severe cases may make it difficult to move around and perform daily tasks.

- **Healthcare cost**: The financial strain and cost of healthcare are increased by frequent medical visits, treatments, and hospital stays.

## The Value of Prompt Diagnosis

It's critical to diagnose BP early because:

**Prevents Complications**: Prompt therapy can shield against severe blistering, scarring, and recurrent infections.

**Improves Prognosis**: Better management and symptom remission are frequently the outcome of early intervention.

- **Reduces Healthcare Costs**: By lowering the need for lengthy therapies and hospital stays, prompt diagnosis and treatment can save long-term healthcare costs.

## Objectives of This Work

This guide's main objectives are to:

- **Educate**: Give thorough explanations of BP's causes, symptoms, diagnosis, and course of treatment.

- **Empower**: Give patients, carers, and medical professionals the skills they need to properly control blood pressure.

- **Support**: Provide tools and techniques for assisting those impacted by blood pressure in managing their condition.

- **Advocate**: Spread the word and push for improved medical research, therapies, and regulations.

## Overview of the Main Ideas

- **BP Definition**: A disease of the immune system that results in big, fluid-filled blisters.

- **Epidemiology**: More prevalent in older persons, prevalence rising in Western nations.

**Awareness**: Essential for prompt diagnosis, efficient treatment, and better results for patients.

- **Misconceptions**: Age exclusivity and contagiousness are two prevalent fallacies.

- **Types**: Multiple forms, such as mucous membrane, localized, and generalized blood pressure.

- **Quality of Life**: Considerably impacted by obstacles related to finances, emotions, and physical health.

* Early Diagnosis**: Crucial to a better prognosis and avoidance of problems.

- **Objectives**: Inform, empower, encourage, and speak up on behalf of BP victims.

## How to Utilise This Manual

This manual is designed to give readers a comprehensive grasp of business processes, covering everything from definitions to in-depth talks about support and management:

- **Start with Basics**: To understand the foundations of BP, start with the definition and summary.

- **Explore Details**: Go further into particular parts to learn more about the types, history, and effects.

- **Apply Knowledge**: Make use of the helpful tips and techniques offered to manage symptoms and enhance quality of life.

- **Seek assistance**: Make use of the links and networks of assistance that are mentioned throughout the guide.

- **Remain Current**: Stay up to date on the latest findings and therapies in the developing field of dermatology.

# CHAPTER 2

## COMPREHENDING THE ILLNESS

### The structure of the skin:

Understanding skin anatomy is the first step towards understanding the Bullous Pemphigoid. The outside layer of skin is called the epidermis, the intermediate layer is called the dermis, and the inner layer is called the hypodermis. Keratinocytes, which are cells found in the epidermis, are essential for preserving the integrity of the skin's barrier and its integrity. Blood arteries, nerves, hair follicles, and immune cells are all found in the dermis. This intricate structure creates a barrier that guards against physical harm and infections from the outside.

## Mechanisms of Immunity:

In bullous pemphigoid disease, an autoimmune condition, the skin's proteins are wrongly attacked by the immune system, causing blisters to form. The generation of autoantibodies, particularly against two proteins, BP180 (sometimes referred to as collagen XVII) and BP230, is a key component of autoimmune processes. The hemidesmosomes, which are crucial for preserving the adhesion between the epidermis and dermis, are the target of these autoantibodies. When these attachments are disrupted, blisters and skin irritation develop.

## The Bullous Pemphigoid's Pathophysiology

Bullous pemphigoid pathogenesis entails a complicated interaction between inflammatory mediators and immune cells. T lymphocytes and B lymphocytes are examples of activated immune cells that penetrate the skin and release cytokines that promote inflammation.

The generation of autoantibodies against BP180 and BP230 is sparked by this immune response. Blister formation and the separation of the epidermis from the dermis are caused by the autoantibodies' disruption of the hemidesmosomes' normal activity.

## Autoantibodies' Role:

Bullous pemphigoid autoantibodies specifically target two skin proteins, BP180 and BP230. These autoantibodies, which are mainly of the IgG type, target the BP180 NC16A domain and the BP230 C-terminal domain. Autoantibodies attach to these proteins and cause inflammatory reactions and complement cascade activation, which exacerbates tissue damage and blister development.

## Influencers of Bullous Pemphigoid:

Bullous Pemphigoid can be caused by or made worse by several circumstances, such as:

1. **Medications:** In vulnerable individuals, some medications, including diuretics, antibiotics, and anti-inflammatory drugs, can cause Bullous Pemphigoid.

2. **Infections:** Bullous pemphigoid disease has been linked to the emergence of infections, especially viral respiratory infections.

3. **UV Radiation:** Bullous Pemphigoid lesions that are already present can get worse by sun exposure and UV radiation.

4. **Trauma:** Patients with Bullous Pemphigoid may develop new blisters as a result of physical trauma or skin injuries.

## Hereditary Propensity:

While there is evidence of a hereditary susceptibility, Bullous Pemphigoid is not exclusively a genetic condition. Some genetic differences may make people more prone to autoimmune diseases such as Bullous Pemphigoid Syndrome. But environmental cues also play a big part in the disease's development, thus genetic factors alone are not enough to cause it.

## Influential Environment:

Environmental variables can affect how Bullous Pemphigoid develops and progresses, such as exposure to specific drugs, infections, and UV light. Furthermore, lifestyle choices like stress and smoking can weaken the immune system and cause illness flare-ups.

## Regular Triggers and Risk Elements:

Bullous pemphigoid is frequently triggered by advanced age (it typically affects those over 60), specific drugs (such as diuretics and antibiotics), a history of other inflammatory disorders, and a hereditary susceptibility. Environmental variables that might cause or worsen the illness include infections and UV exposure.

## Progression of Disease:

Usually, bullous pemphigoid disease develops gradually, beginning with red, itchy skin lesions that may eventually turn into tight blisters. These blisters frequently appear on the flexural areas, extremities, and trunk. There may be phases of remission and exacerbation along the unpredictable course of the disease. Severe blistering and skin erosions could happen, which would be extremely morbid.

## Difficulties and Outlook:

Skin infections, scarring, and reduced quality of life as a result of itching, pain, and deformity are among the complications associated with bullous pemphigoid. Age, the severity of the disease, the patient's reaction to treatment, and the existence of comorbidities are some of the variables that affect prognosis. Many patients achieve symptom alleviation and disease control with proper management, which includes immunosuppressive medicine and wound care. To avoid relapses, Bullous Pemphigoid, however, can be chronic and necessitate long-term care. To control issues and improve results, regular observation and follow-up are crucial.

# CHAPTER 3

## SIGNS AND EXPRESSION OF THE ILLNESS

Bullous Pemphigoid Essential Guide: Symptoms and Clinical Presentation

Bullous pemphigoid (BP) is a long-term autoimmune skin condition marked by enormous blisters (bullae) filled with fluid. Comprehending its clinical manifestation is essential for prompt diagnosis and efficient treatment. Here, we explore the numerous facets of the clinical presentation of BP, offering in-depth explanations of its indications and symptoms.

## Initial Signs and Symptoms

Bullous pemphigoid frequently exhibits non-specific early symptoms that are easily confused with those of other dermatological disorders. Early signs and symptoms consist of:

- **Red, itchy rashes**: Patients frequently experience extremely itchy, red, inflammatory regions of skin before the formation of blisters.

- **Erythema and urticaria**: Some individuals experience hives or diffuse redness, which might be mistaken for common skin disorders or allergic reactions.

## Blister Appearance

The formation of big, tight blisters is the distinguishing feature of BP. Important traits consist of:

- **Tense and fluid-filled**: The blisters are usually large (diameters up to several centimeters), contain clear fluid, and are difficult to break.

- **Firm to the touch**: BP blisters are less prone to break after minor trauma, in contrast to the more delicate pemphigus vulgaris blisters.

- **Hemorrhagic or severe content**: Depending on the intensity and location, the blister fluid may be mixed with blood (hemorrhagic) or clear (serious).

## Lesions' Distribution

One crucial component of the diagnosis of BP is the distribution of lesions:

- **Flexural areas**: The inner thighs, groin, axillae, and lower abdomen are popular locations for blisters to develop.

- **Generalised distribution**: Blisters may, in extreme circumstances, extend to the trunk and limbs of the body.

- **Localised areas**: Blisters may only appear in certain places on a patient, like the lower legs.

# Soreness and Unease

One common aspect of BP is pruritus, or itching, which can have a major negative effect on quality of life:

- **Intense itching**: Patients frequently experience excruciating itching even before the formation of blisters, which may occur weeks or months before any visible changes to the skin become apparent.

**Associated discomfort**: Scratching can worsen the illness by causing secondary infections. Itching can also lead to scratching.

# Mucosal Involvement

Blood pressure can affect mucous membranes, albeit it is less frequent than in pemphigus vulgaris:

- **Oral lesions**: Blisters in the mouth can cause discomfort and make it difficult for a patient to swallow or eat.

- **Other mucosal sites**: In rare cases, blood pressure can also impact the mucous membranes in the genitalia, anus, and eyes (conjunctiva).

## Symptom Variability

Patients' presentations of blood pressure can differ greatly from one another:

 **moderate to severe**: While some individuals may only have localized, moderate symptoms, others may have a serious illness that spreads throughout their body.

**Chronic or relapsing**: Long-term management of blood pressure can be difficult because the condition can have a chronic course with phases of exacerbation and remission.

- **Age-related differences**: Although younger individuals may present differently and may have a more aggressive condition, BP primarily affects the elderly.

## Unusual Demonstrations

Atypical BP variations can make diagnosis difficult:

 - **Nonspecific dermatitis**: Patients without visible blisters may exhibit nonspecific eczematous dermatitis.

- **Crusty or erosive lesions**: Blisters may burst, resulting in ulcers, erosions, or crusts.

- **Dyshidrosiform pemphigoid**: This variation resembles dyshidrosis (pompholyx) in that it causes blisters on the palms and soles.

## Differential Diagnoses

Differentiating BP from other blistering illnesses is necessary for an accurate diagnosis:

- **Pemphigus vulgaris**: Distinguished by a propensity for mucosal involvement and more brittle blisters.

- **Dermatitis herpetiformis**: Usually affecting the elbows, knees, and buttocks, this condition presents as clustered, itchy blisters.

- **Bullous drug eruptions**: blisters brought on by medication that resemble blood pressure.

- **Epidermolysis bullosa acquisita**: An uncommon ailment characterized by distinct underlying pathophysiology but comparable clinical characteristics.

## Observing Symptoms

Sustained symptom observation is necessary for efficient treatment:

**Regular dermatological assessments**: Consult a dermatologist regularly to determine the severity and scope of the condition.

**Patient diaries**: Documenting symptoms, triggers, and treatment reactions can aid in the customization of therapy.

**Laboratory tests**: Skin biopsies to evaluate disease activity and blood tests to track autoimmune markers and inflammation.

## When to Get Medical Assistance

For difficulties to be avoided, prompt medical intervention is essential:

- **Severe blistering or broad rash**: If a significant portion of the skin is impacted, prompt medical assistance is required.

- **Infection signs**: Fever, pus, redness, or warmth could be signs of a subsequent bacterial infection.

- **Difficulty breathing or swallowing**: An immediate assessment is necessary if mucosal involvement affects the respiratory tract or throat.

- **Persistent or worsening symptoms**: Consult a doctor if your symptoms do not go better or if you start experiencing new ones.

Comprehending the various ways in which bullous pemphigoid manifests itself aids in prompt diagnosis and efficient treatment, eventually enhancing patient outcomes and quality of life.

# CHAPTER 4

## IDENTIFICATION AND ASSESSMENT

## Preliminary Clinical Evaluation

**Overview:**

The autoimmune blistering disease known as bullous pemphigoid (BP) mainly affects the elderly. The initial clinical assessment, which includes a thorough history-taking and physical examination, is critical for identifying prospective patients.

Important Points:

- **Patient History:** Compile detailed information regarding the beginning, course, and resolution of symptoms, as well as any possible triggers. Ask about pruritus, which is the itching that frequently occurs before blister formation.

- **Medical History:** Look for any history of drugs, autoimmune disorders, or previous skin issues.

- **Family History:** Look for any instances of blistering or autoimmune illnesses in your family.

**Symptom Description:** Take note of the lesions' appearance, location, and features (blisters, urticarial plaques), as well as any accompanying pain or itching.

# Examination of the Dermatology

**Overview:**

To distinguish BP from other disorders that are comparable to it and to identify its distinctive symptoms, a comprehensive dermatological examination is necessary.

Important Points:

- **Lesion Characteristics:** On normal or erythematous skin, BP usually manifests as big, tight blisters. Usually packed with a transparent fluid, blisters are difficult to break.

**Distribution:** The lower belly, thighs, forearms, and flexural areas are common places for lesions to manifest. Although uncommon, mucosal involvement can happen.

- **Urticarial Plaques:** In the early stages, there may be extremely itchy urticarial plaques without blisters.

- **Secondary Features:** Examine afflicted regions for excoriations or secondary infections.

## Methods for Skin Biopsies

**Overview:**

A crucial diagnostic technique for BP is skin biopsy, which enables immunofluorescence and histological investigations.

Important Points:

Select the biopsy site by taking a sample from a newly formed blister or from perilesional skin, which is the skin that is next to a blister but not directly involved.

- **Procedure:** Employ a punch biopsy technique, usually with a diameter of 3–4 mm, making sure that the depth is sufficient to include the dermis and epidermis.

**Sample Handling:** Divide the biopsy into two specimens: one should be fixed in formalin for routine histopathology, and the other should be placed in Michel's medium or carried fresh for direct immunofluorescence.

# Direct Fluorescence In Situ (DIF)

**Overview:**

For BP diagnosis, DIF is the gold standard for identifying immune deposits in the skin.

Important Points:

-       **Technique:**        Fluorescence-tagged antibodies are used to evaluate a skin biopsy taken from the perilesional region.

**Results:** IgG and C3 are deposited linearly along the basement membrane zone (BMZ) in BP.

**Interpretation:** Positive DIF results help distinguish BP from other bullous disorders by providing solid evidence for a diagnosis.

# Immunofluorescence Indirect (IIF)

**Overview:**

Autoantibodies that are circulating in the patient's serum are found using IIF.

Important Points:

- **Technique:** A fluorescently labeled secondary antibody is used to detect the results of incubating the patient's serum with a substrate (often normal human skin or skin split in half).

**Results:** Circulating IgG autoantibodies against BP antigens (BP180 and BP230) validate the presence of BP.

**Sensitivity:** IIF can still offer useful diagnostic information, but it is less sensitive than DIF.

## Additional Serological Tests and ELISA

**Overview:**

The precise identification and measurement of BP autoantibodies in serum is accomplished by the enzyme-linked immunosorbent test (ELISA).

Important Points:

- **Targets:** Autoantibodies against BP180 and BP230 can be found using ELISA kits.

- **Procedure:** Antigen-coated wells are used to incubate serum samples, and then enzyme-labeled secondary antibodies are used to detect the reaction by producing a discernible color change.

**Interpretation:** High concentrations of particular autoantibodies help confirm a BP diagnosis and help track the course of the illness.

# Distinctive Identification

**Overview:**

To guarantee the right course of treatment, it is essential to distinguish BP from other blistering conditions.

Important Points:

- **Pemphigus Vulgaris:** characterized by mucosal involvement and flaccid blisters; intercellular IgG deposition is seen in DIF.

- **Dermatitis Herpetiformis:** Granular IgA deposits are visible at the dermal papillae in DIF; clustered vesicles are present on extensor surfaces.

**Epidermolysis Bullosa Acquisita:** Blisters and scarring caused by trauma are present; DIF has linear IgG at the BMZ that is comparable to BP but has a distinct antigen target.

# Histopathology's Function

**Overview:**

Important information about the structural alterations in BP is provided by the histopathological analysis of skin biopsies.

Important Points:

- **Tissue Changes:** Subepidermal blistering with an inflammatory infiltrate consisting of neutrophils, lymphocytes, and eosinophils is commonly observed in BP.

- **Subepidermal Blistering:** The dermis and epidermis separate from one another.

**Inflammatory Infiltrate:** One of the main indicators of BP is the presence of eosinophils.

# Tracking Illness Activity

**Overview:**

To evaluate the effectiveness of treatment and the course of the condition, regular monitoring is required.

Important Points:

- **Clinical Assessment:** Monitor the quantity and size of newly formed blisters, the intensity of pruritus, and the general state of your skin.

- **Serological Tests:** Regularly assess autoantibody levels to determine the degree of disease activity (using ELISA).

**Treatment Adjustments:** Adjust medication by patient response and disease activity.

# Recheck and Follow-up

**Overview:**

Maintaining blood pressure and averting relapses require constant monitoring.

 Important Points:

**Regular Visits:** After the disease stabilizes, schedule initial follow-ups often, then sporadically thereafter.

- **Assessment:** Review therapy side effects, symptoms, and skin lesions.

- **Long-term Management:** Modify treatment regimens for the long term, maybe reducing immunosuppressive medication as needed.

- **Patient Education:** Inform patients about the significance of adhering to their treatment plan and how to spot early indicators of relapse.

Bullous pemphigoid patients can be effectively managed and treated by healthcare practitioners through the integration of comprehensive initial evaluations, detailed dermatological examinations, improved diagnostic procedures, and watchful follow-up management.

# CHAPTER 5

## OPTIONS FOR TREATMENT

Bullous pemphigoid is an autoimmune blistering illness that mainly strikes the elderly. It is a chronic condition. A thorough awareness of the available treatment choices and the customization of these strategies to meet the specific needs of each patient are essential for the effective management of this ailment. A thorough reference to the several bullous pemphigoid treatment options is provided below.

## Synopsis of Treatment Objectives

The following are the main objectives of treating bullous pemphigoid:

1. **Control Symptoms**: Reduce scorching, itching, and soreness.

2. **Decrease Inflammation**: Cut down on the immunological reaction that is producing the illness.

3. **Promote Healing**: Help blisters that are already there heal and stop new ones from forming.

4. **Improve Quality of existence**: Make certain the patient can live a decent existence.

5. **Minimise Side Effects**: To lessen negative effects, use the least harmful regimen that works.

## Corticosteroids: Topical and Systemic

Corticosteroids in the System

For mild to severe bullous pemphigoid, systemic corticosteroids—like prednisone—are the mainstay of therapy. They function by inhibiting the immune system and lowering inflammation.

**Benefits**:

- Quick symptom relief.

- Good at preventing the formation of blisters.

**Consequences**:

- Prolonged use may have serious adverse consequences, such as diabetes, hypertension, osteoporosis, and an increased risk of infection.

### Corticosteroids Topical

In mild to moderate cases, topical corticosteroids like clobetasol propionate are frequently used; in severe cases, they are commonly combined with systemic steroids.

**Benefits**:

Less systemic side effects when compared to corticosteroids taken orally.

- Beneficial for small lesions.

**Consequences**:

- The potential for inflammation and thinning of the local skin.

- Less successful in treating widespread illness.

# Agents Immunosuppressive

Corticosteroids are taken with immunosuppressive medications to minimize dosage and negative effects. Azathioprine, methotrexate, mycophenolate mofetil, and cyclophosphamide are examples of common agents.

**Benefits**:

Permit effects of corticosteroids to be spared.

- Successful in preserving the control of disease.

**Consequences**:

- An elevated infection risk.

- Possibility of bone marrow suppression, liver toxicity, and other negative consequences.

# Antimicrobials and Antibiotics

Antibiotics with anti-inflammatory qualities, including tetracyclines (minocycline, doxycycline), may be helpful in the treatment of bullous pemphigoid.

**Benefits**:

- Less adverse effects than corticosteroids and immunosuppressants, with anti-inflammatory benefits.

Beneficial as an adjuvant therapy or in mild to moderate situations.

**Consequences**:

- Disorders of the digestive system.

- The potential for resistance to antibiotics.

# Biological Treatments

Particular immune system components are the target of biological agents. In bullous pemphigoid, rituximab, an anti-CD20 monoclonal antibody, is the most often prescribed biologic.

**Benefits**:

- Targeted treatment with an extended remission period.

- Benefits refractory situations well.

**Consequences**:

- Expensive.

- Potential for infusion responses and serious infections.

# Handling Adverse Reactions

It's critical to control the side effects of treatment well. This comprises:

- Frequent assessment of bone density, blood pressure, and blood sugar.

- Preventive steps, like taking supplements of calcium and vitamin D to avoid osteoporosis.

- Infection control measures, such as immunizations and preventative antibiotic use.

- Frequent lab testing and follow-ups to check for drug toxicity.

## Plasmapheresis's Function

In severe, refractory cases, plasmapheresis, which involves removing antibodies from the blood, may be utilized.

**Benefits**:

- A sharp decline of autoantibodies in circulation.

- Has synergistic effects when paired with other medicines.


**Consequences**:

- An invasive method.

- Needs a lot of resources and numerous sessions.

- The possibility of side effects like bleeding and infections.

# New and Emerging Therapies

New therapies for bullous pemphigoid are still being researched. New treatments consist of:


- **JAK inhibitors**: Focusing on particular immune response pathways.

- **BTK inhibitors**: Preventing signaling from B-cell receptors.

- **Complement inhibitors**: Blocking the complement system from being activated.

**Benefits**:

Possibility of safer and more efficient treatment choices.

- Targeted processes could lessen adverse consequences.

**Consequences**:

Minimal long-term safety information.

- Expensive and difficult to reach.

# Complementary and Integrative Medicine

In addition to traditional therapy, complementary therapies can enhance general health.

- **Diet and Nutrition**: Diets low in inflammation could help alleviate symptoms.

**Stress Management**: Methods like mindfulness, yoga, and meditation can help reduce stress, which can aggravate symptoms.

- **Herbal Remedies**: Aloe vera and turmeric are two examples of herbs that have anti-inflammatory qualities. These, however, ought to be used with caution and under medical guidance.

**Benefits**:

- Holistic Treatment methods.

- May enhance general well-being and standard of living.

**Consequences**:

- Insufficient solid scientific proof of effectiveness.

- Possible conflicts with traditional medical interventions.

## Customising Therapy Schedules

Customizing therapy entails adjusting programs according to:

- **Severity of Disease**: Not severe, moderate, or severe.

- **Patient Age and Comorbidities**: Take into account the patient's general health as well as any other medical issues.

**Response to Treatment**: Modifying by the disease's reaction to the first course of treatment.

- **Side Effect Profile**: Reducing side effects by selecting the best possible course of action.

**Patient Preferences**: Making sure that the treatment plan takes the patient's preferences and lifestyle into account.


**Methods for Customisation**:

- The least aggressive therapy that has the best chance of working should be used first.

- Reduce the dosage and adverse effects of individual medications by using combination therapy.

- Regularly review and modify the treatment plan in light of the patient's reaction and the course of the disease.

Healthcare professionals may give a thorough and efficient approach to managing bullous pemphigoid, improving patient outcomes, and enhancing the quality of life by being aware of and utilizing these treatment options.

# CHAPTER 6

## COPING WITH PEMPHIGOID BULLOUS

Crucial Reference for Bullous Pemphigoid

Large, fluid-filled blisters are a common feature of the uncommon, chronic inflammatory skin disease known as bullous pemphigoid disease (BP). Good management calls for a thorough strategy that addresses many facets of day-to-day life. The comprehensive information in this handbook is intended to assist patients and carers in navigating the challenges of managing blood pressure.

## Routines for Daily Skin Care

Sufficient daily skin care is essential for controlling blood pressure and averting recurrent infections. The following are some crucial actions:

- **Gentle Cleaning:** To clean skin without irritating it, use gentle, fragrance-free cleansers.

- **Moistenizing:** To keep the skin moisturized, use hypoallergenic, fragrance-free moisturizers. Ceramide-containing moisturizers can aid in the skin barrier's restoration.

- **Blister Care:** Keep blisters clean and covered to ensure proper care. To prevent infection and additional stress to the blisters, use sterile, non-stick dressings.

- **Avoiding Triggers:** Recognise and steer clear of certain triggers, such as specific materials, detergents, or extremely high or low temperatures, as they could aggravate symptoms.

- **Sun Protection:** To protect the skin from UV radiation, which can aggravate BP, wear protective clothing and broad-spectrum sunscreen.

# Handling Itching and Pain

Common BP symptoms like itching and pain can have a big influence on one's quality of life. Among the management techniques are:

- **Topical Treatments:** Use ointments or lotions containing corticosteroids to lessen irritation and inflammation. Creams containing non-steroidal anti-inflammatory drugs may also be helpful.

- **Medications Taken Orally:** Antihistamines can assist with itching relief. Systemic corticosteroids or immunosuppressants may be recommended in extreme situations.

- **Cool Compresses:** You can temporarily relieve itching and pain by applying cool, moist cloths to the affected regions.

- **Bathing:** Baking soda mixed with bath water or oatmeal baths may relieve inflamed skin.

## Dietary and Nutritional Considerations

A well-balanced diet can help manage blood pressure and is necessary for general health:

- **Anti-Inflammatory Foods:** To help lessen inflammation, include foods high in omega-3 fatty acids (such as walnuts, flaxseeds, and salmon).

- **Hydration:** To keep your skin hydrated and your general health in check, drink lots of water.

**Avoid Allergens:** Recognise and steer clear of foods that could exacerbate allergies or cause flare-ups. Dairy, gluten, and certain preservatives are common allergies.

**Nutritional Supplements:** Take into account supplements that boost immunity and skin health, like zinc and vitamin D. However, see a doctor before beginning any new supplement regimen.

## Handling Flares

Flares can be upsetting and need to be managed right away:

- **Medication Adjustment:** During a flare-up, work with your healthcare practitioner to make any necessary medication adjustments.

**Rest and Stress Management:** Since stress can precipitate or exacerbate flare-ups, make sure you get enough sleep and practice stress-reduction methods like yoga, meditation, or deep breathing.

**Skin Care Adjustments:** When flares up, moisturize more often and stay away from anything that could irritate your skin.

# Psychological and Emotional Assistance

A chronic illness such as blood pressure can have a negative emotional impact:

- **Counselling:** If you're experiencing anxiety, depression, or other emotional difficulties, think about visiting a therapist or counselor.

- **Support Groups:** Participate in BP patient support groups to exchange stories and obtain consolation.

- **Mindfulness and Relaxation:** Techniques like progressive muscle relaxation, mindfulness, and meditation can help reduce stress and enhance mental health.

# Significance of Consistent Monitoring

For BP management to be effective, regular follow-up with healthcare practitioners is essential:

**Monitoring Progress:** Routine examinations make it possible to track the advancement of disease and modify treatment regimens as necessary.

**Identifying Complications:** Prompt identification of possible issues such as infections or unfavorable drug reactions.

**Lab testing:** Regular blood testing to track how drugs are affecting the body and make sure side effects are not happening.

## Modifying Activities and Lifestyle

Changing routines to account for blood pressure can enhance quality of life:

- **Activity Modification:** Adjust your physical routine to prevent skin injuries. Walking and swimming are examples of low-impact exercises that can be helpful.

- **Adaptive Clothing:** To reduce skin irritation, wear soft, loose-fitting clothing made of natural fibers.

**Energy Conservation:** To avoid weariness, balance activity with rest periods.

## Resources and Support Systems

Making use of the resources at hand can offer helpful support:

- **Healthcare Team:** Collaborate closely with primary care physicians, immunologists, and dermatologists as part of a multidisciplinary team.

- **Community Resources:** For further information and assistance, make use of online resources, patient advocacy groups, and community health services.

- **Financial support:** If you require financial support for prescription drugs or other treatments, look into your alternatives.

#### Patient Advocacy and Education

For BP patients, advocacy and education are empowering:

- **Remain Updated:** Stay abreast of developments in BP research and treatment alternatives.

- **Speak Up for Yourself:** Be honest and upfront in discussing your wants and worries with your healthcare professionals.

- **Educational Materials:** To gain a better understanding of your condition and available treatments, use educational materials from reliable sources.

#### Extended Prospects

Planning and managing BP can be made easier with an understanding of the long-term outlook:

- **Chronic Nature:** Blood pressure is usually a chronic illness that may need ongoing care.

**Remission Possibility:** Many individuals can experience remission, in which case their symptoms either completely disappear or drastically diminish, with the right care.

**Ongoing Care:** To keep the disease under control and avoid relapses, treatment strategies may need to be adjusted and monitored throughout life.

People with Bullous Pemphigoid can effectively manage their condition and retain a higher quality of life by adhering to our detailed guidance. Effective BP treatment necessitates regular meetings with healthcare specialists, appropriate skin care, and access to supportive resources.

# CHAPTER 7

## PARTICULAR POPULATIONS TO BE AWARE OF

Childhood Bullous Pemphigoid:

- Bullous pemphigoid in children is uncommon but can happen; it usually affects teens or those between the ages of 2-4.

- Because of the unusual presentation and little awareness among pediatricians, diagnosis might be difficult.

- Under strict pediatric dermatology care, treatment may include systemic immunosuppressants or topical corticosteroids.

2. **Students with Bullous Pemphigoid:**

Bullous pemphigoid, which frequently manifests as severe blistering and itching, is more common among the elderly.

- Medication interactions and other age-related illnesses may confound the diagnosis.

Treatment should take the patient's fragility, possible medication combinations, and general health into account.


3. **Women Who Are Expectant or Nursing:**

Pregnancy-related bullous pemphigoid necessitates cautious management to strike a balance between the safety of the fetus and the mother.

- Systemic alternatives are carefully chosen with consideration for potential dangers, whereas topical therapies are favored.

- Under medical supervision, breastfeeding can be maintained with the right medication changes.

4. **Concomitant Conditions in Patients:**

- Bullous Pemphigoid frequently coexists with other illnesses such as autoimmune disorders, diabetes, and cardiovascular ailments.

- The effects on general health and possible combinations with current medications must be taken into account in treatment regimens.

5. **Immunely Compromised Individuals:**

- Bullous pemphigoid in patients with impaired immune systems might be more severe and difficult to treat.

The key is close observation and a multidisciplinary team approach including immunologists, dermatologists, and other experts.

6. **Modifications to Treatment for Particular Populations:**

- For unique populations, individualized treatment approaches that take into account factors like age, pregnancy, comorbidities, and immunological state are crucial.

- Medication choices, dosage modifications, and monitoring schedules have to be customized for every patient.

7. **Attention to Paediatrics:**

- Compared to adult cases, children with bullous pemphigoid may exhibit different clinical characteristics and therapeutic outcomes.

- Paediatric dermatologists are essential in providing a precise diagnosis and care that is suited to the needs of the child.

8. **Differences Between the Genders in Management and Presentation:**

- Although both sexes are affected by bullous pemphigoid, some research points to differences in the way the illness manifests and responds to therapy.

- Long-term management plans, treatment outcomes, and illness severity may all be impacted by gender-specific characteristics.

9. **Social and Cultural Aspects:**

Socioeconomic status and cultural values may have an impact on disease outcomes, treatment adherence, and access to healthcare.

- Culturally competent care, support services, and patient education are essential for the best possible outcome.

10. **Personalised Methods of Care:**

- Personalised care takes into account each patient's particular attributes, such as age, gender, comorbidities, and cultural background.

Personalized care plans, frequent check-ins, and patient education all contribute to improved results and a higher standard of living.

## Let's explore some of these subjects in more detail:

Children with bullous pemphigoid disease (BP) are rare cases of autoimmune blistering disorders that usually appear in adolescence or between the ages of two and four. Although BP is more common in older persons, diagnosing and treating it in youngsters poses special difficulties. Atypical clinical characteristics of pediatric blood pressure sometimes include solitary vesicles without noticeable bullae or the absence of pruritus. Therefore, pediatricians who may not be experienced with this illness may misdiagnose or ignore BP.

Histopathological analysis of skin biopsies, direct and indirect immunofluorescence studies, and serological testing for BP autoantibodies are among the diagnostic methods for BP in children. However, because of things like potentially variable test sensitivity and restricted sample availability, getting accurate results from these tests in youngsters might be more difficult.

Children's BP treatment generally follows adult guidelines, but it also necessitates careful consideration of age-appropriate therapy and possible pharmaceutical adverse effects. For small lesions, topical corticosteroids are frequently the initial line of treatment; however, for larger or more resistant lesions, systemic corticosteroids or other immunosuppressive medications may be required. To guarantee proper diagnosis, adequate therapy, and monitoring of potential adverse effects—especially in younger patients—close collaboration between pediatric dermatologists, pediatricians, and immunologists is important.

Bullous pemphigoid affects people of both sexes, however, there are some noticeable distinctions in how the disease manifests and is treated in the two. Research has indicated that women may experience blood pressure slightly more frequently than men, while the reasons behind this gender difference are not entirely clear.

According to certain research, when it comes to clinical presentation, women with BP may show more extensive involvement and a more severe condition than men. Gender differences may also exist in the way that certain treatments, particularly immunosuppressive medication, are responded to. For example, the effectiveness or side effect profiles of some drugs, like corticosteroids or immunomodulators, which are frequently used to control blood pressure, may differ in boys and females.

It's critical to comprehend these gender-specific subtleties to maximize therapeutic outcomes and reduce side effects. When creating treatment regimens for patients with Bullous Pemphigoid, dermatologists and other healthcare professionals should take into account potential gender-related aspects in addition to specific patient traits, preferences, and any pertinent comorbidities.

Now that we have addressed the immunological and genetic components of Bullous Pemphigoid (BP), let's concentrate on how they influence the course of the disease and how best to treat it:

# Genetic Elements

1. **HLA Associations:** A higher risk of having BP has been linked to specific human leukocyte antigen (HLA) alleles. For instance, in several populations, the HLA-DQB1*0301 and HLA-DQB1*0402 alleles have been connected to BP vulnerability. Comprehending these genetic inclinations can facilitate the evaluation of risk and possibly provide insights for tailored preventive interventions.

2. **Genetic variations:** Certain genetic variations and polymorphisms linked to BP etiology have been found through genome-wide association studies (GWAS). The development and severity of the disease may be influenced by these polymorphisms, which may also affect autoantibody synthesis, immune response pathways, and skin barrier integrity.

3. **Familial Cases:** Although the majority of BP cases are sporadic, there have been reports of familial clustering of BP, which in certain circumstances suggests a hereditary component. Inheritable variables and familial disease patterns are clarified through the study of familial instances, which supports genetic counseling and early detection techniques for people who are at risk.

## Elements of Immunology:

1. **Autoantibodies:** The primary indicator of BP is the existence of autoantibodies directed against proteins like BP230 (dystonin) and BP180 (collagen XVII), which are involved in the dermal-epidermal junction. Tissue injury and immune-mediated blistering are caused by these autoantibodies. Treatment choices and disease surveillance are informed by the quantification of autoantibody titers and an understanding of their pathogenicity.

2. **Inflammatory Mediators:** Complement activation and cytokines (e.g., IL-1, IL-6, and TNF-alpha) are examples of inflammatory mediators that, in addition to autoantibodies, are important in the pathophysiology of blood pressure. Research focuses on modifying inflammatory pathways by using immunomodulators or targeted medicines to control blood pressure and prevent illness flare-ups.

3. **Immune Dysregulation:** Both innate and adaptive immune responses are involved in the immunological dysregulation that characterizes BP. Tissue inflammation and autoimmunity are exacerbated by T cell, B, and antigen-presenting cell dysfunction. Comprehending these immunological pathways facilitates the creation of innovative immunotherapies and customized treatment plans.

4. **Environmental Triggers:** Although immunological and genetic factors predispose people to BP, environmental triggers including infections, UV radiation, and drugs (such as dipeptidyl peptidase-4 inhibitors) can aggravate or hasten the beginning of the disease. To manage and prevent disease, it is critical to identify and reduce these triggers.

Precision medicine techniques in BP are enhanced by the integration of immunological profiling, genetic testing, and personalized risk stratification. Researchers, geneticists, immunologists, and dermatologists work together to improve personalized treatment plans for BP patients and get a better knowledge of the disease's intricate etiology.

# CHAPTER 8

## FUTURE PROSPECTS FOR RESEARCH

### Recent Trends in Research

Examining how immune system dysregulation contributes to the development of bullous pemphigoid.

- Examining the possible connection between the onset of the illness and specific drugs.

- Researching how environmental variables affect the development and course of disease.

### Progress in the Understanding of Pathophysiology

- Deciphering how autoantibodies, immune cells, and skin proteins interact in bullous pemphigoid disease.

- Determining the main molecular mechanisms that cause tissue damage and blister formation.

Analyzing how inflammatory mediators influence the course of disease.

## New Methods for Diagnosis**:

By using cutting-edge imaging techniques like reflectance confocal microscopy, blister formation can be seen in real-time.

Investigating the application of biomarkers in skin or blood samples to enable precise and timely diagnosis.

- Including artificial intelligence techniques to analyze histopathology findings automatically.

## Creation of Novel Therapies**:

Examining the effectiveness of biologic medicines with a specific target on blocking immunological pathways linked to bullous pemphigoid.

Investigating how gene editing technologies might be used to control immune responses and lessen the severity of disease.

- Assessing new topical formulations for the targeted treatment of inflammation and blistering.

# Genomics and Genetics' Role

Determining the genetic variations linked to an elevated risk of developing bullous pemphigoid syndrome.

Analyzing gene expression profiles in the skin that are impacted to identify the underlying molecular pathways.

Examining patterns of heredity and familial clustering in various populations.

# Scientific Research

- Calculating the incidence and prevalence rates of bullous pemphigoid worldwide.

Examining regional differences in the manifestation and intensity of illness.

Evaluating the cost of controlling the condition and the amount of healthcare that is used.

# Medical Studies and Trials

- Carrying out randomized controlled trials to assess new treatments' safety and effectiveness.

- Conducting multicenter studies to evaluate treatment response variability and long-term results.

- Working together to create patient-centered research procedures with groups that advocate for patients.

# Databases and Patient Registries

- Creating extensive registries to gather information on the clinical, therapeutic, and demographic characteristics of people with bullous pemphigoid.

- Integrating electronic health records to make post-marketing surveillance and the creation of real-world evidence easier.

- Supporting programs for data sharing to improve data transparency and research collaboration.

# Upcoming Difficulties and Possibilities

- Attending to the requirement for individualized treatment plans based on patient-specific variables and illness subtypes.

- Removing obstacles that prevent underprivileged groups from receiving specialized care and a prompt diagnosis.

- Making use of digital health technologies for patient education, telemedicine consultations, and remote monitoring.

ncouraging Research Participation from Patients**:

- Including patients and carers in the design, planning, and execution phases of research projects.

- Raising public awareness of research projects and clinical trial opportunities via patient advocacy channels.

- Ensuring patient confidentiality, informed consent, and ethical standards in all research involving human subjects.

# CHAPTER 9

## CASE STUDIES AND FIRSTHAND ACCOUNTS

### Case Study: Prompt Diagnosis and Intervention

Providing a case study on the early detection and treatment of bullous pemphigoid can help highlight the significance of promptly identifying symptoms and starting the right medical measures. This could entail talking about the patient's medical background, clinical condition, results of diagnostic testing (such as immunofluorescence and skin biopsies), and the efficacy of corticosteroids and immunosuppressants as early therapy methods.

### Case Study: Handling Serious Situations

Analyzing a case study on the treatment of severe bullous pemphigoid patients will help to illustrate the difficulties encountered and the methods used to control the illness. Aggressive treatment methods, interdisciplinary care coordination, long-term management strategies, and monitoring for possible consequences are a few examples of this.

## Life with Bullous Pemphigoid: A Patient's Story

Understanding a patient's individual experience with bullous pemphigoid may help one better understand the psychological, social, and physical elements of having this illness. Coping strategies, treatment compliance, effects on day-to-day activities, and the value of support networks can all be covered.

## Speech with a Skin Specialist

Speaking with a dermatologist who specializes in bullous pemphigoid can provide knowledgeable insights about diagnosis, available treatments, current research developments, and difficulties encountered in clinical practice. It can also offer helpful advice to both patients and healthcare professionals.

## Nursing Specialist Interview

It is possible to gain insight into the nursing perspective—which includes patient education, wound care management, medication adherence support, and collaboration with other healthcare professionals—by speaking with a nurse specialist who has expertise in caring for bullous pemphigoid patients.

## Case Study: Bullous Pemphigoid in Children

The special factors in identifying and treating bullous pemphigoid in children, such as age-appropriate therapies, psychological support for young patients, and long-term follow-up care, can be discussed by looking into a case study on the issue.

## Case Study: Managing Elderly Patients

Personalized care plans, medication changes, carer engagement, age-related problems, and the management of bullous pemphigoid in older patients can all be discussed by focusing on a case study.

## Perspectives of Carers

Emphasizing the viewpoints of carers helps highlight the vital role that carers play in helping patients with bullous pemphigoid syndrome. This could include difficulties faced by carers, coping mechanisms, interactions with medical professionals, and the effect on carer wellbeing.

## Takeaways from Clinical Experiences

Healthcare workers, carers, and patients themselves can all benefit from thinking back on the lessons they've learned from patient experiences. This can involve strengthening support networks, developing resilience, educating patients better, and streamlining treatment procedures.

## Inspiring Narratives of Overcoming Obstacles

Giving hope, inspiration, and support to those going through similar hardships can be achieved by sharing inspirational tales of people who have triumphed over obstacles posed by bullying pemphigoid. These tales can emphasize fortitude, tenacity, and the value of having an optimistic outlook when managing long-term illnesses.

Each of these components adds to our understanding of bullous pemphigoid, which includes social, emotional, and medical dimensions. It produces a comprehensive manual that helps all those engaged in managing this condition—physicians, patients, carers, and the larger community.

# CHAPTER 10

## USEFUL RESOURCES AND TOOLS

## Symptom Monitoring Records

Logs for recording symptoms are crucial for the management of bullous pemphigoid. Details about the development and intensity of blisters, itching, redness, and any other symptoms you encounter should all be included in these logs. To consistently record these details, you can utilize digital apps or physical diaries. Together with your healthcare team, you can use this information to track changes in your condition over time and modify your treatment plan as necessary.

# Tips for Managing Medication

Taking medicine for bullous pemphigoid requires heeding some important advice. Never miss a dose of your prescriptions; always take them as directed by your doctor. Maintain a list of all the medications you take, together with their dosages and schedules, and consult your healthcare professional about it frequently. Drugs should be stored correctly, and kept out of heat and moisture, and unused or expired medication should be disposed of carefully.

# Checklists for Preparing for Medical Visits

For treatment planning and communication to be successful, getting ready for medical appointments is essential. Make a list of questions concerning your symptoms, the efficacy of your medications, any adverse effects you're experiencing, and any worries you have regarding your health. To aid your doctor in better understanding your condition, bring along your medication list, symptom tracking diaries, and any pertinent medical records.

## Plans of Action for Emergencies

The procedures to follow in the event of a significant flare-up of bullous pemphigoid or other medical emergencies are outlined in an emergency action plan. Provide the phone numbers of your local hospitals, emergency services, and medical team. Make a list of any drugs, such as painkillers or oral corticosteroids, that you could require in an emergency. Ensure that carers or family members are aware of this plan and how to help you in an emergency.

## Suggested Skin Care Products

It's essential to select the correct skin care products when dealing with bullous pemphigoid. To keep your skin clear and moisturized, use gentle, fragrance-free soaps and moisturizers. Products with harsh chemicals or irritants should be avoided. Products like emollients and mild cleansers that are customized to your skin's needs might be suggested by your dermatologist.

## Guidelines for Home Care

A big part of managing bullous pemphigoid is home care. As directed by your physician, take care of your wounds by gently cleaning them and changing their dressings. Use sunscreen and wear protective clothes to shield your skin from prolonged sun exposure. To support your general well-being, maintain a healthy lifestyle that includes a balanced diet, frequent exercise, and enough sleep.

# Advice on Handling Outbursts

Bullous pemphigoid flares can be difficult to control, but following some advice can be helpful. During flare-ups, apply cool compresses to reduce discomfort and itching. Blisters should not be picked or scratched to avoid infection. During flares, heed your doctor's advice on medication adjustments, such as temporarily raising the dosage of oral corticosteroids.

# Techniques for Communicating with Healthcare Professionals

Having good contact with your medical professionals is essential to effectively control bullous pemphigoid. Talk candidly about your symptoms, how well you're adhering to your treatment, and any worries or inquiries you may have. To retain crucial information during appointments, make notes and ask questions when you don't understand anything. Maintain a proactive approach to your health and follow up as advised.

## Building a Network of Support

Having a robust support system will help you during your bullous pemphigoid journey both emotionally and practically. Seek out assistance from loved ones, close friends, and online communities or support groups for those facing comparable circumstances. Talk about your experiences, ask for guidance, and show support to people going through similar difficulties. Your general well-being can be improved and stress can be decreased by having a support system.

## Remaining Up to Date and Informed

Keep abreast of bullous pemphigoid by following developments in the field's research, care approaches, and therapeutic approaches. Participate in instructional webinars, seminars, or workshops about autoimmune skin conditions. For trustworthy information, stick to respected sources like medical publications, associations like the National Eczema Association, and dependable healthcare websites. To receive updates on your condition and make changes to your treatment plan, stay in contact with your healthcare team.

By using these tools and resources, you can enhance your quality of life and manage bullous pemphigoid more skillfully. To make sure that these tactics are in line with your present needs and objectives, evaluate and update them regularly with your healthcare providers.